Summary

Of

The Real Anthony Fauci:

Bill Gates, Big Pharma, and the Global War on Democracy and Public Health (Children's Health Defense)

By

Robert F. Kennedy Jr.

Daniel Tracy

Copyright©2021 Daniel Tracy

All Rights Reserved

The Real Anthony Fauci reveals how "America's Doctor" got his start in the early days of the AIDS crisis by working with pharmaceutical firms to demolish safe and effective off-patent AIDS treatments.

The Real Anthony Fauci explains how Fauci, Gates, and their ilk use their control of the media, scientific journals, key government and quasi-governmental agencies, global intelligence agencies, and influential scientists and physicians to inundate the public with fearful propaganda about COVID-19 virulence and pathogenesis, as well as stifle debate and censor dissent.

Millions of Americans have been persuaded that Dr. Anthony Fauci is a hero by the mainstream media, which is financed by the pharmaceutical industry.

As director of the National Institute of Allergy and Infectious Diseases (NIAID), Dr. Anthony Fauci oversees the disbursement of $6.1 billion in taxpayer-funded scientific research each year, giving him complete control over the subject, content, and outcome of scientific health research around the world.

After more than a year of meticulous and thorough inquiry, Robert F. Kennedy Jr. discovered a stunning revelation that obliterates media lies about Dr. Fauci...

The Genuine Article Anthony Fauci tells how he got his start in the early days of the AIDS crisis by working with pharmaceutical corporations to destroy safe and effective off-patent AIDS treatments.

The Genuine Article Fauci, Gates, and their cohorts use their control of the media, scientific journals, key government and quasi-governmental agencies, global intelligence agencies, and influential scientists and physicians to inundate the public with fearful propaganda about COVID-19 virulence and pathogenesis, and to stifle debate and censor dissent, according to Anthony Fauci.

Robert F. Kennedy Jr., an environmental activist and attorney, talks about his new book, "The Real Anthony Fauci: Bill Gates, Big Pharma, and the Global War on Democracy and Public Health," which is a must-read for anybody interested in learning more about the behind-the-scenes of this colossal fraud.

We could talk about this book for hours and still barely touch the surface of what's in it, which Kennedy calls a "devastating indictment of Tony Fauci."

In a nutshell, Kennedy describes how Fauci converted the National Institutes of Health into a pharmaceutical breeding ground, thus selling the country to the pharmaceutical industry.

The book is a painstakingly researched chronicle of his career of harming human health and reveals him to be a self-serving con artist.

Fauci has aided the vaccination gold rush.

He met with Bill Gates in the year 2000, who demanded that the NIH work with him on a plan to vaccinate the entire world's population with a battery of new vaccines.

In 2009, the accord was renamed "The Decade of Vaccines," with the goal of mandating vaccines for all adults and children on the planet by 2020.

Fauci has spent decades meddling in people's lives and prioritizing business over public health.

Fauci's management of the HIV epidemic is one of the darkest stains on his record, aside from his role in the COVID pandemic.

Fauci began working as a clinical associate at the Laboratory of Clinical Investigation at the National Institute of Allergy and Infectious Diseases in 1968. (NIAID).

He was named director of the National Institute of Allergy and Infectious Diseases in 1984, the year the HIV virus was discovered, and director of the Office of AIDS Research in 1988.

Fauci based the NIAID on an AIDS drug called AZT, according to Kennedy.

AZT was a commercial triumph, but it was little compared to Pfizer's COVID injectable, which made a killing.

It is estimated that AZT alone has killed 330,000 people.

Overall, there are striking parallels between the AZT incident and the current COVID jab and remdesivir situation.

Fauci has warned against using any COVID-19 preventative or therapeutic that relies on low-cost, generally safe drugs like hydroxychloroquine or ivermectin.

The study was funded by US taxpayers, while drug companies made an estimated $100 billion in a single year from the shots, all while bearing no responsibility for accidents or deaths even as people were pushed to take them.

Every year, Fauci is in charge of a $6.1 billion budget.

Fauci is the highest-paid government employee in the United States. At $400,000 per year, the president earns the second-highest compensation.) The money allocated to the NIAID was expected to be utilized to research and improve American health, as well as to eradicate infectious allergic illnesses and autoimmune diseases.

Instead, under Fauci's watch, the chronic disease epidemic has grown.

Despite the fact that Fauci, Gates, and the Wellcome Trust in the United Kingdom fund 63 percent of all biomedical research worldwide, this is the case.

Fauci has overseen the disbursement of more than $930 billion in research money through the National Institute of Allergy and Infectious Diseases during the course of his career (NIAID).

Consider the following illustration: Something happened in 1989 that triggered a chain reaction of epidemics, including autism, food allergies, Tourette's Syndrome, narcolepsy, ADD/ADHD, speech and language impairments, rheumatoid arthritis, and autoimmune conditions such as juvenile diabetes.

They all began around the year 1989.

Why?

What is the root of the issue?

Vaccines, which have increased dramatically since 1989, and virtually all of the chronic diseases that have increased are included as top suspects in the manufacturer's instructions as potential side effects.

Kennedy goes on to explain why Fauci has gotten so powerful in the pharmaceutical sector and how he represents Big Pharma.

Fauci's soiled image and shady history are coming up with him.

When more of Fauci's lies and support of horrific experiments on animals and aborted newborns come to light, Kenney feels he will be forced to resign, especially after the book is released and people learn what he's been up to all these years.

On November 4, 2021, Sen. Rand Paul may question Fauci in front of Congress to back up

Kennedy's prediction that Fauci will be forced to resign.

The comments, which virtually universally attack Fauci, are even more amazing.

In his book, Kennedy included a chapter detailing some of the animal trials that Fauci helped fund.

He also tells a much more horrifying story of Black and Hispanic children being used as guinea pigs.

Fauci recruited these children by arranging for foster children in New York and six other states to be assigned to pharmacological research after their parents died of AIDS.

These children were taking part in illicit research because they lacked a guardian.

Fauci did not want this to happen, therefore he allowed the studies to proceed without the involvement of any of the children's legal guardians.

According to Kennedy, the COVID-19 pandemic represents the apex of Fauci's career.

He describes how Fauci was a key role in pandemic planning – not how to prevent one, but how to create one, because infectious disease mortality had decreased to the point that infectious diseases were no longer a top priority.

COVID, like every other epidemic that has been portrayed thus far, has proven to be a complete fraud.

Vaccines have cost billions of dollars over the years.

Made in the USA
Monee, IL
01 December 2021

83655448R00015